One Foot in
Heaven

One Foot in *Heaven*

A Journey of Faith through Cancer

PAMELA SCOTT

Inspiring Voices®
A Service of **Guideposts**

Inspiring Voices books may be ordered through booksellers or by contacting:

Inspiring Voices
1663 Liberty Drive
Bloomington, IN 47403
www.inspiringvoices.com
1-(866) 697-5313

Because of the dynamic nature of the Internet, any web addresses or links contained in this book may have changed since publication and may no longer be valid. The views expressed in this work are solely those of the author and do not necessarily reflect the views of the publisher, and the publisher hereby disclaims any responsibility for them.

Any people depicted in stock imagery provided by Thinkstock are models, and such images are being used for illustrative purposes only.

Certain stock imagery © Thinkstock.

ISBN: 978-1-4624-0750-7 (sc)
ISBN: 978-1-4624-0751-4 (e)

Library of Congress Control Number: 2013950474

Printed in the United States of America.

Inspiring Voices rev. date: 10/01/2013

Introduction

There are no words to express the magnitude of each single soul on earth. Individual value is eternal and priceless. This is a truth learned through a lifetime. I believe one of our greatest human desires is to be known and be loved. I have found this to be especially true with my children and grandchildren, my nieces and nephews. There is so little time in our world today to clarify our beliefs and share what we believe is important to a life well lived. We all have to find our own paths to this knowledge. We frantically pursue happiness, sometimes unaware that being known comes only through sharing our time with others and establishing love relationships that surpass generations and lifetimes.

This little book is my attempt to be intimately known and to reveal to my family and friends some of the truths I have learned. All the thoughts I would like to share with my loved ones are lost in a time warp of current existence. Life is busy and wisdom does not often come into focus unless we take time to pursue the basic questions and listen to our souls. Sitting down with someone we love to exchange wisdom is rare.

My life with cancer has offered me the opportunity to get back in touch with the most significant life issues. Facing death brings new priorities and perspectives. For me, these are the ultimate truths gleaned from years of living. Through a life of making mistakes, following wrong paths, and fostering self-centered attitudes, I have come out of the darkness and into the light of gratitude, sharing time, loving unconditionally, and coming to terms with mortality. The content of my stories and the life-giving sustenance they have brought to my own life may, in some way, offer something good to someone else—a lifeline, perhaps, or a new form of guidance. This is my hope. This is my reason for wanting to be known.

CHAPTER 1

One Foot in Heaven

She said you know what heaven is like?
& I said I wasn't sure & she laughed
& said grown-ups didn't know much at all
about important stuff & I said I had to agree with her
even though I was one of them myself.

—BRIAN ANDREAS

ROM BIRTH TO DEATH, EVERY human being has one foot in Heaven. The Heavenly foot keeps us aimed toward goodness and love. The earthly foot keeps us grounded in earthly concerns. On our best days, life is a good gift. On our worst days, it is a veil of tears. I believe that life is meant as a practice ground for getting love right. It takes a lifetime to learn that love is in its highest form only when it is unconditional. It also takes a lifetime to realize that the knowledge of death is our reminder to make the most of the time we are given. I've never been to Heaven, but my pages of earth have a Heavenly margin. I see Heaven in people, especially in children. I see Heaven in nature, especially in the stars. I see Heaven in God's rainbow. I see Heaven in the random acts of kindness humans do for one another—sometimes not so random. My capacity for love has grown since I turned toward Heaven.

I knew a woman once who was close to death. I wanted to talk to her about her feelings and fears. She would not believe she was dying. Her faith never wavered. She believed that God would heal her before death came. He took her home to Heaven anyway, which is a form of healing, but I felt bereft that we never talked about such an important event in her life and in mine. I took from the sadness a belief that when my time came, I would share the insights I could gather in the hopes of alleviating some of my own fear and leaving behind a thread to follow.

I received my cancer diagnosis two days before my sixtieth birthday on December 22, 2004. That day has changed the way I look at life and death. Life is no longer something I take for granted. I have come to the realization that I have lived my life unconsciously, waking for brief moments of clarity and thoughtfulness but returning to a sort of stupor.

Consciousness teaches us how little we truly know. Those who would have us plan our lives from beginning to end surround us in our society. Take charge, set goals, redefine self, and take care of number one. Though it is all good to a point, this plan doesn't include those things that control us, such as illness seems to want to do. To discover a mission and a purpose for a fulfilling life, sometimes we have to listen to what our souls are saying. That ember inside each of us, which reflects the light of God, is our guide. God is in the fine points, though I often forget to notice Him.

When I think of God, I think of a masculine and feminine spirit. If I leave out either aspect, there is not the balanced depth to God's mind. To consider God as male or female is to diminish spiritual understanding. He made both male and female in His image, and so for me, God is the great I AM.

It is easy for me to get a glimpse of God's spiritual love by watching a beloved dog named Sammy. Many domesticated animals give us all their love without condition, without reserve. When I think of a joyful heart, I remember Sammy waiting patiently for his mistress, my friend, to come through her patio gate. He looks to her for a toss of the beloved, bedraggled toy that sends him bounding from one end of the room to the other, only to repeat the play until both are exhausted. The bountiful joy of animals, especially dogs, gives us a picture of God's heart toward us. Any attention toward Him, no matter how small, gives our God joy. My belief in God has given me strength to surmount obstacles that ordinarily would have destroyed me. Cancer has been one of those devastating experiences in my life.

Whether I pray in gratitude or supplication, I can transform my mind. I have found that peace comes from love and gratitude, despite the worst of circumstances.

CHAPTER 2

Heavenly Hope

Signs like these will accompany those
who have professed their Faith;
they will use my name to expel demons,
they will speak entirely new languages,
they will be able to drink deadly poison without harm ...

—MARK 16:17–18

*K*NOWING ABOUT MY CANCER FILLED me with unspeakable fear. All the horror stories I had heard about cancer came flashing back in sickening detail. I had recently heard a celebrity tell of her experience with chemotherapy. She told her audience that she thought she would surely die. I cried to my husband that I didn't think I could go through with this treatment. I was wrong. It may sound crazy, but even with the loss of my hair and nails, I never felt I was going to die, at least not from the chemo.

Nurses and doctors were constantly checking my status to relieve me of any negative symptoms. I felt surrounded by love and support. After searching the Web and every other source I could find, I concluded that cancer was not necessarily a death sentence, not yet anyway. During this crucial time, God reassured me through my friends and loved ones.

Despite the circumstances, my husband and I decided to celebrate my birthday with a party. We both needed the diversion. He made his famous chili, and I invited my friends who didn't have anywhere to go on Christmas Eve. We didn't talk about my cancer news; we just had fun. It was the first party I remember in years, and it was filled with lots of love and underlying encouragement. I look back on that Christmas Eve as a turning point for my future months and years.

On January 11, 2005, the day of my mastectomy, as I entered the hospital, I looked up to see a statue of our Lady, Mary, above the front door. Her grace surrounded and comforted me as I faced the fateful day that I would lose a precious part of my body. I have been looking up ever since, and I truly believe I am still alive because I sacrificed that body part—and because I am not finished with my earthly mission.

My husband and I felt comfort by the presence of five of my

book club friends, Jeanne, Joanne, Eleanor, Joy, and Barbara, who sat waiting with him for news about my surgery at Providence Hospital in Everett, Washington.

I had a regular habit of attending morning Mass. I had a very special friend who knew a woman diagnosed with breast cancer, and she wanted me to meet her. The meeting hadn't happened yet. But this particular morning, I sat next to an unfamiliar face. After Mass, my friend Jeanne, who was sitting behind us, joyfully introduced me to the unknown woman. The stranger's words stilled my fears. Sadly, I don't remember her name, but I remember what she said. She told me that she was a fourteen-year survivor of breast cancer. I asked her what she did, and her simple words were, "I did everything the doctor said."

She also said that something had told her to "get out of bed and come to Mass that day." She convinced me that God sent her to me, because I know from personal experience that is how He sometimes communicates with me. I have not seen her since, but she gave me the gift of hope.

Love poured in and over time, I found my focus there instead of on the disease. The women in my neighborhood gave me a basket of special items to comfort me: a purple pillow for my naps, an icepack eye cover, a box of chamomile tea, sweet-smelling cards full of loving thoughts and prayers, and a CD that one neighbor remembered as my favorite. The music of *Air Supply* became a symbol of the supply of love I received from my neighbors at a time when I was desperate. Every time I listen to the CD, it brings back that love. These same women also set up a dinner night for every scheduled chemotherapy day during my infusion stage. My husband and I had eaten better during those chemo evenings than we had in the previous fourteen years of our marriage.

At the time, I had been working at a Ben Franklin Arts and Crafts store, one of the few left in the country. My friends at work made me a quilt with family pictures they had gleaned from a Christmas calendar I had made that year. Their surprise cheered me on, and I still cover up with the quilt, feeling its softness and love on my down days. Remembering all the love is what truly keeps me going and the love keeps coming. I am conscious of its healing properties and I take them into my soul. I know they are sent directly from God through His faithful.

Another divine intervention was the morning in Mass when I heard the introductory scripture that begins this chapter. Though I thought I had listened to all the scriptures, I had not been conscious of this one until that day. I have held fast to this scripture because I truly believed that chemotherapy was poison, and when I read the consent form, I felt like walking away. Why would anyone want to take this stuff despite its ability to kill the cancer? I was sure it would kill me.

We had a priest, Father Dan, who taught scripture as if he had experienced it with every detail. I truly loved him. After Mass, he called the Mass participants to the altar to put their hands on me, and he gave me a healing blessing with holy oil. The memory of that moment has been a constant reminder that it's not over until God says it's over and by then I know He will have made me ready.

I firmly believe these events set the tone for my future. There are those who would say that God does not intervene. I believe He sends His angels with messages to others so that they carry out His will. If any one of them had not been listening, perhaps my own outcome would not have been the same.

My year of cancer went by very fast. Before I went through radiation therapy, I traveled to Houston to see my newborn granddaughter, Sophia. I owned my life again and felt a sense of accomplishment at having come through the treatments. While I was undergoing radiation, my nephews from Michigan and Hawaii came to visit. Their presence gave me another boost to beat the cancer.

They filled my hours and days with something much stronger than the disease itself. Their love and caring concern gave me the strength to survive.

After a month of daily radiation, I was finished. My hair came back curly, and though I never would have chosen the style for myself, it looked good. My energy returned and all my fears were put to rest. In retrospect, I realize that my fears were so much worse than the reality. It is not easy for me to say, but losing a breast was a small price to pay for the life I saved. As I look back on that year, I have forgotten my chemotherapy side effects; what I remember most is the love.

My cancer years have been different from my other life. Though I went into remission for almost five years, eventually the cancer returned in my bones and liver. Cancer changed me. After I developed cancer, I noticed the love more often. Time does not stop, though I thought it might, but the changes cancer made in my consciousness helped me accept it with an element of grace. I am a survivor, and I want to encourage anyone facing this disease to know that we are made of stronger stuff than we can ever imagine. I did not want to become a victim, and I fought to keep the disease from taking over my life. Eight years into this, I am still winning my emotional battle most of the time.

CHAPTER 3

Heaven on Earth

Our birth is but a sleep and a forgetting:
The soul that rises with us, our life's star,
Hath elsewhere its setting,
And cometh from afar;
Not in entire forgetfulness. And not in utter nakedness,
But trailing clouds of glory do we come
From God, who is our home.

—WILLIAM WORDSWORTH

$\mathcal{I}$'VE NEVER BEEN TO HEAVEN, but earth supplies all I need to know about Heaven. Wordsworth's poem expresses the idea that we are born with Heaven in us. Heaven is in our children. As our childhood feet become more accustomed to earth, we grow further from the inner spark that is our source. The thread that joins us to God becomes invisible and hard to imagine. We begin to suffer separation pains. Slowly we grow and settle into our lives on earth, but we never totally lose that spark that draws us slowly back to the knowledge of Heaven, the knowledge that God exists.

My favorite work of art is of an elderly, bearded angel who stands in a window looking out. The work is by Paul Wilson titled *Earthbound,* and it speaks to me. We are bound to earth for a time as we make our way back to Heaven. Our lifetime earthly journey provides glimpses of Heaven as we carry out our mission. It is a journey fraught with danger, and the knowledge of evil invades our Heavenly space. It wasn't supposed to be this way, but freewill caught us in a moment of profound error, and we surrendered to the desire to know evil as well as good. Love and gratitude for life as we know it is the only way to reestablish our Heavenly connection, and it takes many of us a lifetime to return to God's all-encompassing love.

Heaven informs our mysteries on earth. One night, I was driving down a dark deserted road in Gilbert, Arizona. There were no streetlights or houses near the road. A stop sign loomed in my headlights, and so I stopped. My windows were down. No sound, not even a cricket sounded the alarm, but something inside of me told me to be still. Out of the darkness, I heard an echo getting closer. As I waited, searching the dark road to the left, a car with no visible headlights sped through my intersection at possibly ninety miles an hour. Following in chase was a black and white police patrol car with no siren or headlights. As the two cars disappeared into the night, I realized that if I had pulled forward from the stop sign, both vehicles would have smashed into my driver's side. I have often wondered what influenced me to stop and wait. It is a mystery not easily resolved, and yet, the experience has made life more precious. When I was first diagnosed with cancer, I did extensive research to discover what I did to cause cancer to grow in my body. "Maybe it was ..." became my mantra. I felt frenzied to find answers and yet over time, I realized there were no answers. Sometimes it's genetic and uncontrollable. Why I developed cancer is a mystery to me.

Medical research has come a long way in providing answers to my questions, but they seem to change as more is learned. One thing that hasn't changed is the pharmaceuticals used in cancer treatment are easier on patients than they used to be. When I look around the infusion room, I see so many loving nurses and patients who are determined to project a positive attitude. I believe we are all in this together and it gives us the hope we need to get through. Some days a harpist comes and plays for us. One time during my infusion, I received a foot massage. There are so many who want to help. The nurses are kind and efficient. I believe that these men and women are gifts from a loving God who inspires them to love us through the process of illness.

I have always believed in Heaven, but since I have been on my cancer journey, I look for reasons to support those beliefs. I notice more blessings on earth that give me a glimpse of Heaven. I need to believe that color is a Heavenly gift to my soul, born in the freedom and mystery of individual truth because it is evidence of something more. I believe our souls brought the appreciation of color with us when we were born. Color tells me quite a lot about Heaven, and in my opinion, is one of the most important earthbound glimpses of creation. The colors of the peoples of civilization reveal the earthen rainbow of humanity who promises that life will continue.

The greatest proof for the existence of God is the circle of life. When a child is conceived, there are no words to express the magnitude of that one single soul. There is no way to communicate the greatness within that tiny re-creation of life. That God entrusts the responsibility of that soul's journey to our human imperfection boggles my mind.

I believe that raising children is our greatest challenge and our greatest mission. Raising children is also the greatest achievement that exists. No matter what is written, constructed, or imagined, nothing compares to one child who grows up to bring love to this world.

I see Heaven in the colors of nature as it accentuates the beauty of our world. Color is mysterious and offers secret significance to the essence of my consciousness. It evidences a magnificent realm, unimaginable to my mind. My memory can reproduce color so that I can hear it and smell it. I hear blue in the rush of waves toward the shore. If I close my eyes, the smell of the beach can arouse a vision of the color of sand or the gray of a whale squirting her salute as she passes along her watery highway to the sea. I hear green in the whispering pines swaying overhead in the spirit of the forest teased by the breezes originating from that illusive wind.

God's rainbow is important because it reflects Heavenly promises. I remember the line in the 1985 movie *The Color Purple* where Shug Avery says, "I think it pisses God off when you walk by the color purple in a field and don't notice it." Its subtlety begs us to notice that it is natural evidence of God's love for us and as such, provides the sunbeams and the shadows that point to Heaven. The grandeur of color is a clue to the magnificence of creation and its eternal secrets.

Color inspires the human soul and instills desire to capture art on canvas, explore nature, or sit on a beach and watch the waves splash toward the shore. Through color, humanity often recognizes that life has a grander origin than we may ever understand, and we respond spiritually to its influence of archetypal knowledge with innate gratitude.

Color can feed the inner yearnings of a spirit in search of hope, light, splendor, and virtue. During my chemotherapy treatments, I found intent in the genius of the golden sun to nourish my life on earth. I sat in the sun often and felt its healing power. I believe that the effect of the azure sky gave strength to my weary soul, and that God predetermined its blessing since the beginning of life. Color is nature's emotion. There is purpose in the power of a white rose to instill peace in the midst of inner conflict. The green of rebirth instills in the heart of humanity the recognition that nature's continuous encore revitalizes itself, heedless of the struggle.

Life with cancer can go through the cycle of rebirth in much the same way. As the hair grows back, we are blessed with new awareness. Judging from my conversations with others, many cancer patients feel the same. Nature's green inspires humanity to complete the cycle of inner rebirth, again and again despite challenges and with conviction. Color is the essence of life, from the skin tones of humanity to the azure of the sea and sky, God is telling us His story—that we all belong to Him, that He loves us, and that life is eternal.

For me, life also has a mystical element that we cannot ignore in our quest for truth. It is this knowledge that has enriched my own life through many years and given me strength of my inner spirit, sensed though unproved. I have discovered Heaven on this earth. We are often skeptical of those ideas or theories which we cannot prove of our inner or outer universe. We are suspicious of dreams and miracles because we are unable to explain their origins or their irregularity.

Ordinarily, I do not remember dreams. After I married my second husband, I found myself still deeply influenced by my previous marriage. There were memories of my former relationship

I simply could not avoid. I knew my emotional baggage influenced the success of my new relationship, but I could not stifle the thoughts and regrets.

In the dream, my first husband sought to rekindle our relationship. Habits and traditions of twenty years of marriage were a powerful lure in his direction. I dreamed of the relationship I now had with my current husband. In my dream, I could not leave the safety and security of his love for me and mine for him. My dream gave me insight and resolved my conflict. The feelings in the dream were so authentic it was as though I had lived the decision in that precise moment and made a choice based on something beyond my own understanding. I have been grateful for that new awareness that stilled my doubts and allowed me to go forward in my life. It had a great influence on my belief in the power of inner forces I do not understand. For me, that silent thread connected to God is slowly returning to my consciousness preparing me for my return to Heaven.

One day, I faced a particularly fear-filled dilemma. I had just moved to a new town, had no money, and could not find a job. I made the decision to sell my car in the hopes of getting my finances under control, but knew without a car, I would not have transportation to the illusive job I needed. I had heard a minister talk about expecting a miracle, so I turned my hopes toward that idea. Soon the phone rang, and though I did not understand how it worked, the ability to talk to someone miles away through a machine on the wall, revealed a miracle to me. Later, I was vacuuming and once again, I perceived a silent knowing that this technology was miraculous. Later in the day, I found a backyard garden, left by a previous tenant, and I pulled up a carrot. It slowly dawned on me that miracles filled my life though I had not recognized them. I'm not sure what miracle I expected, but I gained something so much more important. I discovered that life is a miracle and that so much of what we have comes from sources beyond our understanding while we struggle to believe that we have total control.

I did not sell my car, but I did find a job and the lesson that I took away from that miraculous day lives on in my memory as a great gift—childish enthusiasms, perhaps. Though our logical minds will certainly credit my vacuum cleaner and telephone to man's earthly development, there are mysterious elements to each of them. Carrots need sun and rain, both of which lie far beyond our abilities to produce. Man's knowledge and control is made possible through invisible realms and universal mysteries that can never be explained except by the existence of a power beyond us.

A Christian would say that these insights come from God. The world we inhabit is stirred by spiritual manifestations of the Virgin Mary of Medjugorje and the role of angels in our lives. We have listened to and read of men, women, and children who have died and gone to Heaven only to return to our world with tales of the afterlife sharing stories of fascinating lights and long-dead ancestors who inspire and strengthen our human spirit. Stories of medical healing, miracles, and saving graces through prayer confound our imagination and provide divine coincidences of remarkable and illogical events. How is it possible to synchronize these impressions with logical belief systems when they are unexplainable? I believe the prayers of my friends and family and even people I didn't know have bought me time, just as my treatments have bought me time to appreciate my life and learn to live with a grateful heart.

For me, these secrets of our universe add an enchantment to the workings of my imagination toward creation, and as such, give texture and mystery to my life on earth. I find less significance in knowing from whence our mysteries come than in knowing that they do come to give us sustenance, courage, moral foundation, and the ability to arrive at unconditional love, gratitude, and ultimate sacrifice. Whether it was the potential of my brain or angel whispers,

I am alive today because I listened to a voice or a thought inside myself, which gave me a direction that saved my life. I recognized a fulfilling relationship because a decision was made in a dream that influenced my well-being.

The mysteries of life are all intertwined in the truth that is experienced by each individual human soul. Though we continuously question, there is profundity to our existence, which we cannot analyze or shelve in neat categories of fact. Life's unique and awesome quality makes it fascinating. Revelation progressing slowly from a world understood through religion and science, working together to ponder mystery, makes perfect sense.

CHAPTER 4

Building Bridges

The Bridge Builder

An old man going along life's way
Came at the evening cold and gray
To a chasm, vast, and deep and wide
Through which was flowing a sullen tide.
The old man crossed in the twilight dim
The sullen stream held no fears for him
But he turned when safe on the other side
And built a bridge to span the tide.

"Old man," said a fellow pilgrim near
"You're wasting your strength with building here.
You've crossed this chasm deep and wide.
Why build you a bridge at evening tide?"

The builder lifted his old gray head
"Good friend, in the path I've come," he said,
"There follows after me today
A youth whose feet must pass this way.
This chasm that was but naught for me
To that fair-haired youth, might a pitfall be.
He too must cross in the twilight dim.
Good friend, I'm building this bridge for him."

—AUTHOR UNKNOWN

*T*HE CANCER THAT HAS LITERALLY taken over my body has caused me to rethink what is important in my life. Though I place hope and trust in my chemotherapy, I do it with an element of faith. That is a belief that all chemotherapy comes from God's pharmacy. I know that when doctors tell me I may only have six months to live if I don't submit to chemo infusions, the prognosis is serious. Since my breast cancer diagnosis, MRIs, CAT scans, and bone scans have become a way of life and have uncovered new lesions in my bones and new sites invading my liver.

There are days when I live in dreadful fear of the unknown and wonder if I will be brave enough to die gracefully. I wonder what burdens will be placed on my family before I turn toward Heaven for the final time. I find myself wanting to get rid of or finding homes for the possessions I have collected for more than a lifetime. I don't want them to overwhelm my husband after I am gone. I want to leave an understanding of who I am and how much I love them to my grandchildren, Sophia and Noah, who give me such joy. I don't want to say good-bye to my son who has been the center of my world for so long, or to my daughter-in-law whose beauty and spirit I have come to treasure. I can't imagine a life without my husband, who has become my steadfast soldier guarding me through my battle.

These fears sneak in on the days when I am not trying to ignore it all and live in the protection of denial. I have made a pact with myself to build a bridge while I follow my path toward Heaven. I want to leave a thread that will help those who come after me to face the inevitable with profound understanding and lack of fear. I want to leave courage to share the journey toward Heaven for those who might want a guide. I want to share my knowledge of God with those who want to believe that He truly is with us in challenging details.

I do not believe the saying that God never gives us more than we can handle because I don't believe God gives us our troubles and heartaches. I have seen many who have been bombarded with way more than they can handle. God did not intend for us to wander around in an earthly veil of tears.

As I see it, knowing evil is an aftermath of discontent. I tend to overlook my blessings, searching for something just beyond my grasp. I am no different from my biblical parents or our Jewish ancestors who roamed the desert for forty years. I have found that gratitude turns the tide of evil. My Heavenly foot has connected me to the most compelling idea, aside from love, that has crossed my earthly path. Living with a grateful heart has become my goal.

When I am consistent in my appreciation of life in all its manifestations, I am happy. When I find valuable lessons in difficulties and hope in hard times, I feel I am walking in a Heavenly direction and Heaven will help me. It is easy to be grateful for the joys in our lives. It is quite another challenge to be grateful for the sorrows. God does not send us these sorrows, but the act of living does. Sometimes we make our own troubles, sometimes others contribute to our tears, sometimes there is absolutely nowhere to place the blame, but always God will help us if we ask. Eventually, we discover that so much of life is out of our control. God may not do as we ask, but He will do what is best. He may not change the situation, but He will change our understanding of it. We can live gracefully or at odds with the uncontrollable aspect of living. In the beginning, God gave us choice, and so it remains for us to decide how we will live in this world not totally of our own making.

I believe God has the final word. When I have the patience to wait on Him, I am less afraid and more joyful. The dreaded six months have come and gone, and I am still joyfully alive. I did submit to the medical therapies that will slow down the metastasis and buy me time, though fear threatened to overtake me once again.

I find that new discoveries are making the infusions less painful, at least for me, and that medical science is now running toward a cure. I should have already placed my second foot in Heaven by now. I believe I am still here because prayers overpower the disease and give me hope, and because I have a mission in life that I need to complete. The days feel more like a gift when I am not taking them for granted. I continue to look up. I continue to be grateful for every new day.

I don't know how much longer my life will go on. The truth is none of us does. The unknown can be a blessing or a curse. When I look on it as a curse, I feel afraid and give in to giving up and crawling under my bed. When I look on it as a blessing, I take every day to the bank for cash to spend. Because I live in a sort of limbo, I have time to notice nature in her glory and people in their goodness. I pray for every person I see, especially those on the side of the road holding a sign that says God Bless.

There is a spirit within each of us that strives to help us achieve happiness, nowhere more important than in life-sustaining human connections. An example that comes to mind is an incident that happened one day many years ago as I drove past Chandler High School in Chandler, Arizona, after having dropped my son off for school. I don't recall what troubled me, but I still remember feeling bleak and isolated, lonely and unsure. I looked up as I passed a young man, unknown to me and probably my son's age, walking to school. As our eyes connected, he smiled. His smile instantly enlightened the gloom within me. His memorable smile has lasted in my mind for twenty-six years. I never saw that boy again, but I have often wondered if he was an angel put on this earth in that very moment solely to cheer me. I will never know the answer, but I do know this, one of the best things about life is that those divine coincidences can happen anytime, anywhere, and when we are most in need of them.

I remember the day I was driving along a busy street feeling desperately sorry for myself. I looked toward the side of the road to see a man without legs scooting along the gravel on a makeshift rolling board. Was he an angel, probably not, just a man who had been given a cross, and I could see him bearing it with great dignity.

The story of a young boy named Christopher is still vivid in my memory. I worked in a bank located in a shopping mall. As I headed back to the bank from lunch, I saw a young boy, maybe twelve, running along pulling flowerpots from their places and throwing them on the ground. I thought he was just a troublemaker. Minutes later, as I walked out of the mall through a side door, I saw the boy go out another door, oblivious to oncoming traffic. My fast-moving feet stopped abruptly in the middle of the sidewalk almost without my permission. I looked back to see him running wildly toward oncoming cars. I ran to grab him from the parking area, and he followed me without reservation. I sat down with him, and he laid his head on my lap. I realized that something was frightfully wrong. Words came strongly into my mind. *He is diabetic and needs some sugar.* I called to a person in an Orange Julius store nearby, and someone brought me a glass of orange juice and some sugar packets. As I made the young boy drink the juice, someone called an ambulance that eventually took him to a hospital. I went back to my bank. Days later, his sister came to my teller window and waited in line to tell me that her brother had taken an accidental overdose of his insulin shot that day and if I had not helped him, he would not have lived.

Every time I doubt that God exists, I remember Christopher. Each one of us has a story to tell. These kinds of moments in my life don't happen just to me. God is always strumming that invisible Heavenly thread. He sends us experiences that mold us into saints while we remain sinners. God connects our one foot in Heaven with our other foot planted firmly on earth.

CHAPTER 5

Listening to Heaven

No evil shall befall you,
Nor shall affliction come near your tent,
For to his angels he has given command about you,
that they guard you in all your ways.

—PSALM 91:10–11

I CAN USUALLY FORGET THAT MY life is turning the last corner when I am busy with daily tasks. However, when I lay my head on my pillow at night unwanted thoughts bombard my mind. My life flashes before me in endless streams of self-reflection. My fears magnify in the dark. The pains that I ignored in daylight threaten my peace at night. The monster under the bed becomes the voice of doom. I find it hard to trust that everything will work out as it should. I struggle to believe that I will receive whatever grace I need to make the transition from earth to Heaven when the time comes. I think of Jesus in the Garden of Gethsemane praying His last prayers, drops of blood caused by human fear pouring down His face. I am right there with Him. Though I know I belong to Heaven, I am in love with earth. Though I have accepted the inevitable, I find that I really don't want to leave yet. Though I believe in healing miracles, I know that my mission on earth will end.

When I thought I was dying, I literally gave up. With every new lesion, I was convinced I had little time left. It was a spiritual death. I no longer cared about much. I quit my beloved job at a bookstore because I had no strength and was afraid of breaking a bone. I found it impossible to get interested in books of any kind, especially sad ones or ones that evidenced man's inhumanity to man. I quit shopping for clothes because I felt severely overweight with nowhere to go except medical appointments. I couldn't enter into trivial conversations that were meaningless and shallow. I felt the words of the Native American Chief Joseph, who said, "I will fight no more, forever." All the activities that gave me joy were out of reach or gone. I just wanted to get my final exit behind me. I sat in my recliner watching mindless television and waiting to die.

Elisabeth Kübler-Ross says there are stages to our grief and that death is the final stage of growth. I thought I was at the final stage when I accepted my fate, but now I know that acceptance can't mean giving up. I needed to get out of my chair and make a difference until my time had come.

I read somewhere that angels do not have the five senses of sight, sound, smell, taste, and touch in quite the same way as we have them. Angels come to earth to serve God's creation, and they have no need of our human gifts. I'm not sure I would want to be an angel under those circumstances. Hearing my grandchildren laugh, listening to their mother or father read them a story, or watching them play in the backyard, provides happiness in my life. My daughter-in-law has a way of making my son laugh that brings joy to my heart. How could Heaven produce the aroma of a family Thanksgiving meal or the wonderful scent of bread in the oven? How could the sights and sounds of Christmas be matched in a Heavenly realm? Is music as beautiful there? I treasure the touch of my husband's hand or the feel of his cheek on mine. I cherish my friends who help me cope with life and who pray for me unceasingly. I can't imagine life without these earthly riches. New awareness of earth began a transformation in my thinking. I listened to the evangelist, Joel Osteen, who reminded me that I needed to believe I had a future. Reading and listening to his words renewed my hope in a new day. Joel helps me get past my pity parties. He doesn't judge them; sometimes we need them, but too much is unproductive. I get it. Joel's words kept me looking up and believing in a loving Creator.

I am convinced a coincidence of a divine nature inspired my three high school friends from Arizona to come for a visit. Knowing they were coming gave me a reason to go on living a little while longer. Surprisingly, I slowly threw myself into house cleaning, a room at a time, for days, with help from my Washington friends. The familiar activities boosted my spirit, and my anticipation of my friends' visit gave me a reason to live a little longer. I found no time to commiserate on my prognosis nor did I overlook that I was capable of more than my sadness would have me believe.

We had a Heavenly visit. We basked in the sunshine of one another as though we had not been disconnected for twenty-two years. The kindness of my friends brought me back into balance. They left part of their hearts with me, and I passed through my hour of loss because I felt God's presence in my life through them. Through others, God reminds us that He is here with us. The visit from my lifetime friends stabilized my courage. Turning toward Heaven has revealed affluence on earth that I often took for granted. Our lives are composites of joy and sorrow, light and dark, good and evil. I think I have often focused too much toward the dark side and not appreciated all the light that was available to me.

I have no answers as to why God does not intervene in all painful situations. I like to believe that if all of us on earth would listen to our soul's voice, there would be more of our own intervention. My inner voice speaks to me, and I listen more now than I used to, but I still don't listen enough. When I do, the reward is so much greater than I could ever expect.

In Maryland, on my way to teach school each day, I passed a corner where an older man was selling newspapers. One day I had an idea. I pulled my car in to where he stood and without a moment's hesitation bought all his newspapers. The smile that broadened his toothless face was an extraordinary sight. The random act had given him something. What? A reason to hope? A reason to believe? A gift of love? Whatever he felt shone from his eyes. I felt it too. I knew that listening to my spirit had produced for each of us a life-affirming comfort from the soul.

The experience of listening and acting is always the same. I see someone; I feel an urgency to slip them some cash, a grocery gift card, a judgment deferred, or a prayer. I'm not always fully responsive.

One day, I drove around a block because I could not get the idea to give out of my head. I kept hoping I wasn't hearing a message because I didn't want to turn around and go back. Traffic was heavy and I was tired. I saw a man sitting on a curb quite far from the road holding a small sign in his hand. I knew that begging was his intent. I got out of my car and walked toward him. When I handed him some money, he thanked me and asked if he could give me a hug. I said, "Let's just shake hands." I've thought time and time again that I might have missed a hug from Jesus.

CHAPTER 6

All Truths Lead to God

If you live according to my teaching,
You are truly my disciples;
Then you will know the truth
And the truth will set you free.

—JOHN 8:31–32

*T*RUTH HAS BECOME A RARE commodity in our culture. Political candidates tell us what they think we want to know and then they do their own thing. Advertising would have us believe that beauty and happiness are about how we look and what we possess. Media coverage stretches into the realm of absurdity, and we, like frogs, unwittingly and slowly begin to boil in our saucepan without recognizing the need to jump for safety.

I believe that most of us have the common sense to realize that our direction is precarious, but we have neither the means nor the energy to fight against what seems like a majority. The truth is, we are on the road to being lost, and so we may find ourselves turning toward Heaven. Surprisingly, that is not a bad thing.

My own life has been based on faith in God and the intrinsic value of humanity. Faith has been a certain attitude that fosters confidence and reassurance, and gives me a reason to believe that all things in life happen within a framework of existence created by a loving God who is concerned about me. Truth is important to me. When it is tested, I find the need to regroup, reevaluate, and emerge stronger and more certain. Truth comes in brief insights and serendipitous understandings that come from a God who is paying attention to what we need to be successful in our pursuit of unconditional love, which is our mission on earth. The spiritual crisis I experienced with my cancer diagnosis reminded me of another crisis years earlier that threatened my faith.

My return to school at fifty complicated my naive faith. Though my faith has been a firm foundation and strength for me through the years, knowledge temporarily complicated the truths of religion. Though we celebrate Columbus's discovery of America in the name of Christianity, it is also true that Native Americans do not celebrate this holiday. Columbus initiated the slave trade with the capture of his trusting Indian captives. The Puritan ". . . city upon a hill . . ." taken from John Winthrop's 1630 sermon, "A Model of Christian Charity," which became the ideal for New England colonists, described America as God's country, but I'm not sure God was proud of some of their puritanical ways.

In 1963, my innocence was shattered by the revelations of the civil rights movement which sought to make all Americans equal though we were always in God's eyes. The doubts were threatening my peace. I began questioning again. I had come to a spiritual crisis in my life. I needed to find answers that would rebuild the beliefs that kept my spirit turning toward Heaven. Faith in some of our Christian history seemed to crumble beneath my feet.

During my college years, I prayed for truth realizing that I no longer knew the truth and hoping it could set me free. What I found was that freedom came from knowing that the path toward truth always leads to God. I believe with my whole heart that we as a country are still blessed by God. I believe that good will win in these trying times, and America will discover that our majority still believes in God. We may call Him by many names—Allah, Jehovah, Buddha, the Creator or a higher power—He is the God for all worlds, the great "I AM" (Exodus 3:14). The consistency of thought in our world religions supports basic truths consistent with the golden rule of love as spoken by Jesus in the biblical chapter of Luke 6:31, "Do unto others as you would have them do unto you."

As scientific discoveries of life and the world's religions evolve, it seems evident that the people of earth are moving toward the realization that we owe our creation to the same God revealed to us through a unified soul. Embedded in the minds and souls of humanity is the truth that we do not exist for ourselves alone, that life is the ultimate gift, and that the purpose of life is to love. Each religion that has survived has spread similar values and truths and has professed peace and love as the divine achievement of humankind with the reward of eternal life. All great religions walk the road of benevolence, similar in their beliefs. Their diversity merely strengthens what will eventually evolve.

Because of my spiritual crisis, I began to research the beliefs of others whom I respected for their knowledge of the universe and their understanding and abilities to clarify their beliefs. Einstein believed that eventually education confirms faith. Jung believed that faith and knowledge of God were imbedded in human souls since creation, and that from the beginning of time, all civilizations were influenced by what he called his Theory of Archetype, a collective unconscious that informs our soul.

J. R. R. Tolkien had insights that brought the primitive myths to explain the archetypal truth of the ages into the realm of the present. C. S. Lewis struggled with his faith just as I have done and then left behind a legacy of apologetics for Christianity that would surely convince even Satan.

There are spiritual considerations that are intangible yet significant to human existence. My own spiritual experiences convinced me of the mystery reflected in beliefs of John Keats, the romantic poet, who bequeathed us an idea called the Theory of Negative Capability. Keats believed we needed to be comfortable with the mysteries of life without struggling to have all the answers. There is wisdom about John Keats that appeals to my introspective mind because he was facing death at an early age. His letters stand alone as examples of a pure heart on a journey to discovery of life-sustaining thoughts meant to inspire the process of living for whatever time he had left. I am right there with him. I want to spend my days loving and my nights believing that there will be new elements of existence when my own feet walk through that Heavenly gate.

The makeup of our physical bodies amazes me. I believe that the understanding of God's creation thrives on the biological and cosmological details we have learned from science. When I found myself for the second time being prepped for a power port which makes the drawing of blood for lab work and infusions easier on the veins, I was not in a good place. I had been avoiding the inevitable surgery because I knew I never again could be without the port. My surgeon literally bounced into my curtained space reminding me of Tigger in the *Winnie the Pooh* books. He asked me health-related questions such as did I have diabetes or high blood pressure? He named several diseases. I answered no to all of his inquiries, which led him to pronounce cheerfully that I was a very healthy woman. I suppose my face registered a shocked expression because he sheepishly clarified, "except for the cancer."

Surprisingly his opinion triggered gratitude. He was right. My body was protecting me in so many ways, and I realized that my situation could be so much worse. Whenever I walked into the cancer waiting rooms and saw the other patients, some who looked like walking corpses, I reminded myself repeatedly how much worse it could be. However, I've also seen evidence of the triumphant spirit that rises up and meets this disease head-on, transforming the individual back to health. The patients, whose situations seemed hopeless, become inspiring testimonies to the miracle of our body's ability to overcome adversity.

I heard a story once about a chemistry professor who taught at a large university. At the beginning of every semester, he would stand in front of his class and challenge anyone to prove there was a God. He set the tone for class by his atheistic mind-set because no one would stand up to him.

One Christian young man in school, who had heard about this professor, did everything he could to avoid the class. Finally, the time came when he had to take chemistry, and this was the only class available. At the beginning of the semester, the professor stood before the class with his customary challenge, and everyone lowered their gaze waiting for the smug professor to exclaim that if no one could prove the existence of God then he would not hear His name spoken in class. Silently, the young man stood up. The professor smiled at the thought of a chance to make this student look foolish.

"So you think there is a God," the professor said, and the boy nodded. "Well, then prove it."

The professor held up a science laboratory beaker and announced that he would acknowledge the possibility of God if after he dropped the glass on the hard cement floor it failed to break. The boy closed his eyes and spoke an innocent, faith-filled prayer. When he was finished, he nodded for the professor to drop the bottle. With a flourish, the professor dropped the glass object. A collective gasp came from the class as the bottle rolled off the professor's foot and onto the hard surface without breaking. Sheepishly, the professor returned to his desk and the boy sat down. The professor never again uttered his challenge. It has been my experience that God works through natural means, even a soft shoe, to make his presence known.

The scientific ideas of every age lead us closer to God's truth. Darwin's theory of evolution does not negate God. Evolutionary change is inevitable, granted the way our earth was formed. Current ones have replaced earlier theories of our existence, but no theory has disproved the existence of God who spoke the universe out of darkness according to biblical text. It has been written that one of the greatest scientific minds of our times, Carl Sagan, ". . . never understood why anyone would want to separate science, which is just a way of searching for what is true, from what we hold sacred, which are those truths that inspire love and awe." (The Varities of Scientific Experience, pg xi). His argument was not with God, but with our lack of appreciation of what scientific study of the universe, in our own lifetime, has revealed about God through a scientific approach. Without it, our understanding diminishes.

In his television series and companion book *Cosmos*, Sagan proclaimed that we are made of star stuff. I'm happy to know this as a scientific fact. I like the idea. It reminds me of Job 38:4, "Where were you when I laid the foundations of the earth?" I was among the stars waiting for God to infuse me with a soul and send me to earth.

When I think of the complexities within our solar system alone, I am speechless. The intricacies of space boggle the mind. The astronomy class I took on my return to school contributed to an even stronger faith. I found it one of the single, most important demonstrations of God's magnificence I had ever experienced. The words of Abraham Lincoln come to mind, "I can see how it might be possible for a man to look down upon the earth and be an atheist, but I cannot conceive how he could look up into the heavens and say there is no God."

The class had a profound effect on my faith. While I felt myself in sinking sand during that time, the power of the universe to inspire hope gave me a reason to press on toward truth. God was in that Heaven fifteen billion years ago. Only He could have created such majesty.

The conviction that God exists comes from within. My soul knows what it knows because of that invisible thread that trailed behind me at birth and connects me to Heaven. During the Age of Enlightenment, Blaise Pascal believed that "The heart has its reasons of which the reason knows nothing. The heart feels God, not the reason. This is what constitutes Faith."

The path to truth is a long one and it takes a lifetime. We can never let the discouragement of our times cause our apathy. Our history is marked with good and bad decisions by powers of the past. Our current culture is facing some troubling issues in society today, but I believe if we look up we will find our answers, and they will be the right ones. Life's purpose changes with a belief in God. The consistency of thought in our world supports basic truths that have not disproved the existence of God, but have built bridges to new knowledge as we continue to discover our universe. We need not fear. New scientific evidence, born out of truth, always leads to God.

CHAPTER 7

Suffering

I slipped His Fingers, I escaped His feet,
I ran and hid, for Him I feared to meet.
One day I passed Him, fettered on a Tree.
He turned His head, looked and beckoned me.

Neither by speed, nor strength could He prevail.
Each hand and foot was pinioned by a nail.
He could not run and clasp me if He tried,
But with His eye, He bade me reach His side.
For pity's sake thought I, I'll set you free.

Nay—hold this cross,' He said, 'and follow Me.'
'This yolk is easy, this burden light,
Not hard or grievous if you wear it tight.'
So did I follow Him Who could not move,
An uncaught captive in the hands of love.

—FROM *LIFE IS WORTH LIVING* BY FULTON J. SHEEN

J'M NOT SURE WHY GOD doesn't relieve all suffering. Our own free choice is a big part of the mystery. I believe that suffering has the potential for power. If we are Christian, we believe that one man, human and divine, bought back our right to Heaven through unimaginable suffering. When challenged by the opportunity to suffer here on earth, we can use that suffering to share in His suffering. But it doesn't end there. Though we don't look on ourselves as divine, we have divinity within us through our gifts of the Holy Spirit. From our Christian perspective, because of the humanity and divinity of Jesus Christ, holy people like Gandhi, Muhammad, Confucius, the Buddha, or Mother Teresa have been inspired by that divine Holy Spirit sent to us through the life of God on earth. For a Christian, the power of Christ rests with His cross. The Christian believes that God loved humanity so much that He sacrificed His only son to ensure immortality for everyone. Only divinity could encompass so much power, but without His humanity, Jesus could not represent the human race.

The story of all stories is one told by Bishop Fulton J. Sheen who described the essence of the cross and resurrection. A judge, God, was asked to preside over a case of murder. The accused man was brought before the court to receive his sentence. No righteous judge could allow a murderer to go unpunished but the prosecutor could produce no evidence of evil. There was no body lying in the tomb and no proof to substantiate the act. The man on trial was set free because death did not prevail. That man, exemplified by the humanity and divinity of Jesus Christ through the benefit of God's sacrifice and forgiveness, could overcome death and return eternally to Heaven.

I believe that I can use my suffering for the benefit of loved ones. Because of that divinity in me, my suffering can transform a situation or move a soul at risk toward Heaven. Suffering is a powerful prayer for good. In my personal world, I offer my suffering for the good of my son's family, especially my grandchildren. Up to this point, my physical suffering does not compare to my mental and emotional pain. My greatest sadness now is that I live more than a thousand miles from my son and his family and feel a longing to be near them during the time I have left. I offer this up every day, and it gives me a reason to hope that I am making a difference in their future despite my absence in their lives. It helps me to accept and use the heartache and gives me a sense of peace in the midst of my sadness.

I watched an interview once with a young man who had become a Christian as a teenager. When the interviewer asked him how it happened, the boy told this story. He had been in a gang but discovered he wanted to spend his life differently. He tried to extricate himself from the situation but found the gang refused to let him go. They sent him a message at school that they would shoot him as he left the building. His overwhelming fear caused him to remain inside the school. Soon his mother heard of her son's terrifying situation. The boy's mother went to the school, and after some consideration of the problem, walked out of the building with her son putting herself between him and his gang. The amazed boy turned his life around because he realized his mother would sacrifice her life to protect him, and Christ's cross now made sense to him.

An event that will forever live in my memory is the capture of the DC snipers. In October of 2002, I lived in Frederick, Maryland. The shootings occurred intermittently during a three-week period. Residents of the area were shot down while grocery shopping, pumping gas, mowing their lawns, and walking to school. I remember being afraid to leave my home. I found courage in the acts of kindness that brought the gang called the Guardian Angels from New York City to our ravaged, fear-filled towns. These gang members could be seen pumping gas, standing in doorways, and otherwise making their protective presence known. Their unselfish dedication to others is well known in New York, but knowing about them and having them in my vicinity during that horrific time became an everlasting faith builder.

Our country's freedom has been consistently won through the suffering and sacrifice of our nation's military. Like the angels of paradise, they place themselves in harm's way to dispel evil in our world. Just as we see evidence of Heaven on earth, we also see evidence of hell. War is hell. The suffering it causes is a potent reminder that there are those who will suffer for the sake of others. I believe that suffering for others changes lives if offered within the framework of love.

CHAPTER 8

Death

Psalm 23

The Lord is my Shepherd; I shall not want.
He maketh me to lie down in green pastures;
He leadeth me beside the still waters.
He restoreth my soul;
He leadeth me in the paths of righteousness for his name's sake.
Yea, though I walk through the valley of the shadow of death,
I will fear no evil; for thou art with me;
thy rod and thy staff they comfort me.
Thou preparest a table before me in the presence of mine enemies;
thou annointest my head with oil; my cup runneth over.
Surely goodness and mercy shall follow me all the days of my life;
and I will dwell in the house of the Lord forever.

—KING JAMES VERSION

*A*s I'VE GROWN OLDER, I see that life is a tapestry of spiritual threads woven in time. There is so much more than we can ever know. Time alone brings truth into focus, but we must be ready. The truth that stands alone in life or death is love. We search for love, we respond to love, and we grieve when it goes away. The thread of love fulfills. We alone have the power to give and withhold love. I believe I need to give more than withhold. Death gives me the reason to love deeper, stronger, and more unconditionally in life. Death makes me notice how much life means. The knowledge of death makes me want to spend my days in harmony, revealing only love through my actions.

There is no consolation for the death of a loved one. It is the ultimate sorrow. I remember the death of my mother as my first experience with death. Knowing that I had taken her for granted filled me with a deep regret. I vowed never to repeat my mistake. Years later, I lost a high school friend in a plane crash. Once again, death affected my life and confirmed my own mortality. Someday I would die. Once again, I made a vow—this time to be ready. I began to question not just about death but my reasons for being alive. I don't believe we can find our purpose until we begin to ask questions of this magnitude. I found answers that have served me well in the years since. I have looked on these deaths as epiphanies in my own life. I finally understood that there is more to death than loss.

The billions of years of universal existence are beyond our limited knowledge and understanding. Carl Sagan reminded us "Lost somewhere between immensity and eternity is our tiny, planetary home." His thought makes me wonder why our lifetime is so short. How can we know that the quality of our lives on earth is only a preparation for a universal transition to something more?

After these many years, I do not visit the empty shelter of my mother's grave; she does not dwell there. I contemplate the someday when we will meet again, when I will once again fold myself into her arms and feel loved. There will come a day when I will know the truth about death. Until then, I am emotionally bound to this earth and to those who exist in my world. Birth on earth is the beginning of a fascinating journey that is exciting, compelling, difficult, and heartbreaking. Being bogged down in the heartbreak cannot be allowed to obscure the magnificence and the love.

Living one day at a time has been my saving grace. Eternity is such a far away word, such a long way to visit. Life stretches ahead on unknown paths, yet there has to be some purpose. Though death is the end of life as we know it, it is not the end of the journey. Life is a preparation for the mystery to come. The earthly finality and pain of death gives us reason to make the most of life through loving. The immensity of our soul, that connected thread that travels between life and death and between Heaven and earth, is measured by the capacity our spirit has earned through love. Wide or narrow, our loving soul is the spiritual thread woven into our own loom of time returning our feet to Heaven.

Though I have down days, I know they will pass. Though I am hopeful, I am also looking Heavenward. I live in the present now. My favorite T-shirt exclaims Life is Good. Death has taught me to live every day with a grateful heart. Gratitude is a universal truth. It is central to life just as the mathematics of relativity is central to physics and astronomy, just as gravity connects us to earth. Living in gratitude brings God's universal principles into our lives—joy in the midst of sorrow, peace in the midst of pain. Gratitude fosters a consciousness of importance and overlooks triviality. Gratitude repairs resentment, and nurtures unconditional love, our life's mission on earth.

Death does not discriminate. At some point in every life, each of us will understand the mysteries of Heaven. Death is not an end but a beginning. Howard Storm wrote my favorite story of the afterlife in his book, *My Descent into Death*.

In the midst of trauma after his death, he found himself lying on the ground surrounded by hideous creatures gnarling and pulling at him. He heard a voice coming to him that was not his own saying, "Pray to God." He had lived his life essentially atheistic, and even in death he argued with this voice. Finally, after extensive resistance, he responded to the voice and sought his memory for a prayer he might have known in childhood. Mixed with a jumble of childhood songs, he found remnants of the twenty-third psalm. To his surprise, the words antagonized his tormentors, and they screamed obscenities at him while they slowly backed away into the darkness. As his life flashed before him, he realized that most of his time had been spent in courting egoistic illusions. His fear of his present circumstances was elevated by his despair. His narcissism had landed him in the sewer of the universe fighting off demons. He did not believe in life after death and now he found himself in hell.

As he laid there, a song from his innocent childhood and sung in his own voice floated to his consciousness, "Jesus loves me ..." His voice strengthened in an entreaty to Jesus to save him. Time stood still as a radiant light enveloped him. In his words, "This person of blinding glory loved me with overwhelming power." Then, "We rose upward, gradually at first, and then like a rocket we shot out of that dark and detestable hell. We traversed an enormous distance, light years, although very little time elapsed."

Howard's story is amazing, but the awe-inspiring idea for me is that even after death, Heaven is still confronting evil to recover our soul.

Facing cancer has taught me to live with one foot in Heaven. Heaven has taught me how to leave a thread for others to follow. Though I know there will be much more in the end, I am now ready to face whatever comes. The fears have subsided. Gratitude for the life I've had is my treasure. I am thankful for those who have loved me and for those I have loved.

Death is a blank page. Though it comes to all of us, it is on its own mysterious clock. I find that a blessing. When I thought I knew my time, I felt already dead. My fervent prayer has been that I would have time to say good-bye to the people I love. God has honored that prayer. I have been walking slowly through this valley of death. It has given me a new appreciation for life. Most of my fears have abated because of my relationship with my Shepherd who is walking with me. He walks by my side at every step. He sends other walkers who carry His staff to comfort me. He provides a community of Saints on earth to pray for me and keep my Heavenly clouds of glory intact so I can find my way back home when the time comes. His grace is always sufficient to my task. I have felt this in my life but never as extensive as now. I have experienced love in my lifetime but never as potent as now. I have put my past behind me, carrying only its lessons into my present. The future is a hill that stretches before me though I cannot see what is on the other side. The future does not belong to me anymore. It belongs and always did belong to God. Despite my health prognosis, I now know that my life is not over until God says it's over, and I am finally comfortable with that knowledge.

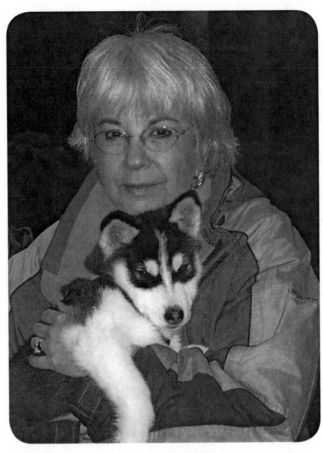

Pamela and Miki

Biography

PAM SCOTT returned to school in later life to become a teacher. In 1999, she earned her degree in English from Sam Houston State University. She has a son and daughter-in-law and two grandchildren, Sophia and Noah, who live in Houston, Texas. She lives with her husband, Mike, in Snohomish, Washington.

In Memoriam

Pam passed away peacefully at home on June 20th, 2013, surrounded by her husband, close and loving friends, and the Angels of the Hospice Team. She is greatly missed and remembered with love. It is my honored privilege to be able to finish the publishing process of her book, "One Foot in Heaven" as I promised her I would. As was her hope, it is also mine that this book will ". . . offer something good to someone else—a lifeline, perhaps, or a new form of guidance." God be with you, Pam. Yours was a life well lived. I'll love you always.

Michael Scott
Pam's loving husband

CPSIA information can be obtained at www.ICGtesting.com
Printed in the USA
BVOW08s1057291013

334931BV00001B/7/P